Baby Mamas

A Midwife's Guide to Ending the Epidemic

Jay Von Muhammad

ISBN: 1-4392-5390-0
ISBN-13: 9781439253908

To order additional copies, please contact us.
BookSurge
www.booksurge.com
1-866-308-6235
orders@booksurge.com

Dedication

This Guide is dedicated to my husband Robert, the love of my life.

Thank you for taking me from Baby Mama to 'Wifey' over 14 years ago.

CONTENTS

Acknowledgements

- God
- The Teachings of the Honorable Elijah Muhammad (NOI)
- My three fabulous children, Desjunae, Nailah and Ji-had.
- Sacramento Birthing Project Clinic. This clinic is providing a service to underserved women in Sacramento that is unparalleled.
- My Best Friends, Beth Jackson, Dadisi Najib, Cynthia Gi, and Cora Stewart.

How to Use This Guide

I began writing Baby Mamas: A Midwife's Guide to Ending the Epidemic, because of my goal and desire to improve the alarming infant mortality rate in the black community. It is my belief that the leading, non-medical, contributing factor to the high infant mortality rate in the black community is the Baby Mama Epidemic (women having babies from men that they are not in relationships with, or not married to). This epidemic, as does a high infant mortality rate, affects the black community disproportionately.

As I continued to write, and through discussion with peers, it became clear that the information in this guide is relevant to all women, regardless of race. Despite it's relevance to all women, many of the references are directed toward black women. Please do not let that discourage you from reading this guide and benefiting from the information provided.

Baby Mamas: A Midwife's Guide to Ending the Epidemic, is full of 'Lessons Learned' from over 10 years of experiences working with pregnant women, and women in general. All of the 'Real Stories' are true, and the information provided comes from hands on experience. It is written in easy to understand terms, and there is no need to have a college reading level.

As you read through this guide you will find that the focus is more about the psycho-social issues (mental and social health) of pregnant women, and less about the physical aspects of prenatal care. There have been countless books written about prenatal care, various prenatal tests, and prenatal procedures, but very few books written about psycho-social issues affecting pregnant women.

Please do not be offended by any of the language in this guide. It is simply a representation of the actual language spoken on the streets by young women and men. I did not include it to be offensive, but I believe that there is no other way to address this problem then by using real terms and scenarios.

As a society, we have been ignoring the Baby Mama Epidemic, and even normalizing it. I wrote this guide because there is NOTHING normal about being a Baby Mama.

This guide should serve as a 'communication piece' in communities throughout the US. It is time that we have honest dialog about the Baby Mama Epidemic and its' impact on society. More importantly, we must answer the question of how the Baby Mama can become the Wife. It is only through dialog and education that we will create healthy mamas, healthy families, healthy babies, and as a result, healthy communities.

INTRODUCTION

I can remember the first time I heard that black babies are almost three times as likely to die as white babies in the United States. There was something very unjust about that statement, and it cut me like a knife.

Why would black babies die more? What is different about black women or black babies? Since internally we are all (generally) the same, it has to be what is happening outside our bodies. Environmental! What we go through mentally and spiritually, in addition to physically.

After more than 10 years of working with pregnant women, I have come up with my own explanations and conclusions about why black babies die more. Not scientific, just obvious. Some things we can change immediately, by changing our behavior, others will take some time because they have become part of the healthcare institution.

Disparities in Healthcare
In the black community, when we use the term Healthcare Disparities, we are referring to the differences in the quality of healthcare, and access to healthcare, between black people and other races. Our argument is that these differences and deficiencies exist because of racism.

Disparities in healthcare contribute to the high infant mortality rate (numbers of babies that die during pregnancy, and shortly after birth) in the black community.

Healthcare Disparities have become a part of the healthcare institution. Some of the obstacles that we will have to address to overcome the disparities in healthcare are racism, lack of culturally competent providers in the black community, environmental injustices, and preconceived notions and judgments about our communities.

Lack of Culturally Competent Healthcare Providers

Historically, there have been trust issues between black people and the healthcare system. Why? One of the driving forces of distrust between black patients and the healthcare system is that blacks have been the victims of medical experiments and medical racism.

Magnifying the trust issues is a lack of culturally competent healthcare providers in the black community. What do I mean by this? Well, patients do better with clinicians who are sensitive to their issues, who have similar backgrounds, look like them, and have an understanding of their customs, culture and traditions. Clinicians need to understand the 'lingo' of their patients. That helps to build the trust.

The lack of culturally competent clinicians is sometimes a deterrent to patients, causing them not to seek medical care. During pregnancy, the result is little, to no prenatal care.

Preconceived Judgments & Racism

Clinicians are just people, and people often make judgments about other people because of ignorance, race, or stereotypes. For instance, I have worked with many doctors who believe that patients who are insured by Medi-Cal are Non Compliant (they don't listen), so they either won't accept them as patients, or they don't get excited when they do.

If your prenatal care provider is not excited about caring for you, you should stop going there right away! Excitement is what makes us good at what we do. It is what makes us go that extra mile. You are worthy of excitement from your clinician.

Lastly, racism is an ugly disease that not only affects other aspects of society, but it affects the healthcare field as well. Although clinicians may deny it, the numbers don't lie. Countless studies have proven that blacks receive a lesser quality of healthcare than whites. This is why culturally competent healthcare providers and having a doctor that looks like *you* is so important.

Lower Socio-Economic Status

Many clinicians are not willing to work in underserved communities. Not only is it not lucrative, but it is difficult. Before they meet you, they have already made a judgment about you. As a midwife, I can understand why some clinicians feel like this. It has been my experience that patients from lower socio-economic backgrounds and communities have complicated cases. In my patient population, these patients are more likely to be involved with drugs in some fashion, either as an abuser, a co-dependent, or a distributor. They also tend to have complicated medical histories and many psycho-social issues (bad relationships, mental health conditions, etc). Not to mention, a lack of support, education and information.

Environmental In-Justice

Black communities have larger amounts of environmental pollutants, be it from power companies and other dangerous plants, racism, or other socio-economic ills.

I am a product of a community that has over 50 "Hot-Spots", and one "Superfund Site." These are areas that are toxic and dangerous to humans because of hazardous chemicals. It is no surprise that this community has the highest infant mortality rate in San Francisco.

This reality is repeated in city after city throughout the United States. Unhealthy communities, producing unhealthy mamas, producing unhealthy babies...A vicious cycle.

The issues that we have just discussed will not be changed over night. Addressing these issues will have to be done through a large public effort. However, the issues that we will discuss in the next chapters can improve immediately if women are willing to change bad behaviors

Chapter 1
Thinking of a Master Plan

If You Don't Have a Plan, You Become a Part of Someone Else's Plan

Black women don't plan pregnancies. Instead, pregnancies are just happening. Oops! As a result, we are merely reacting to the news that we are pregnant. This news is sometimes good, but more times, not so good.

Since we are merely reacting to the news of pregnancy, valuable time has been lost. Some of the most important weeks of pregnancy are the first 12. By eight weeks of pregnancy, a woman has already completed most of her first trimester. The primary development has already occurred, meaning that although the woman may have just learned of the pregnancy, she is already behind.

Not planning for pregnancy leaves us behind! It means that we did not take the necessary precautions before conception, and in the earliest weeks of pregnancy. We did not take Folic Acid, which helps to prevent birth defects, or prenatal vitamins, which provide us, and our babies with critical nutrients. We didn't have the opportunity to take into consideration the use of alcohol, drugs or prescription medicines. Planning pregnancy is extremely important because it allows women the time to prepare, mentally, physically, and spiritually for the creation of their babies.

So Now That You Are Pregnant, Which You Didn't Plan, What You Should Know

The Value of Prenatal Care

Why is prenatal care, or the lack thereof, so important? Because, when you receive the proper prenatal care you begin the process of educating yourself about how to have a healthy baby. The earlier you seek care, the more time you have to learn.

My experience has been that the lower the woman's socio-economic status (the poorer the woman), the less involved she is in her prenatal care. She tends to want the clinician to make all the decisions about her care, instead of seeking her own information and education about procedures, tests, and pregnancy. She wants the clinician to just tell her what will be done to her. This is a recipe for disaster.

I have also noticed that the lower the socio-economic status of the woman, the less the clinician is willing to educate and involve her in her prenatal care. When a clinician cares for a patient who is insured through Medi-Cal, or other State or Federally funded insurances, the clinician receives only a third (or even less) of what they would if they were treating a patient with a PPO insurance. The result manifests in less time educating and empowering the patient, so that the clinician can see more patients in less time. Less time equals less care, less time equals less education and information. The result is an under informed mama, which is a risk to the community in it's' entirety.

In contrast, the patient with the PPO insurance receives a longer visit with more explanations, an opportunity to ask questions, and better deliverance of quality of care. The clinician knows that *this* patient will accept nothing less.

Prenatal Care isn't optimum if you are uninvolved and undereducated. If this is the case, you are a victim and not a participant.

Chapter 2
Ignorance is NOT Bliss

The Hand that Rocks the Cradle Rules the World

As midwives we learn lots about helping women have healthy babies. We tell women all the time...If you want to have a healthy baby you have to eat a nutritious diet... don't do drugs...breastfeed...stay away from stress...and so on...

What I know to be true is:

THERE ARE NO HEALTHY BABIES WITHOUT (FIRST) HEALTHY MAMAS
(mentally, spiritually, and physically).

What do I mean by this?

Well, before I talk to you about having a healthy baby, I have to first identify your obstacles to being a healthy mama. If your life is full of stress, how can you focus on a healthy baby? If you have a drug habit, how can you 'just stop', so you can focus on having a healthy baby? If you are unemployed, or underemployed, how can you buy nutritious foods to eat during your pregnancy so that you can have a healthy baby? If you are in a dysfunctional relationship, how can you give your attention to having a healthy baby? It is nearly impossible!

We are a community of sick women, and most of it is mental…The thoughts we think, our behaviors, our beliefs, and what we find to be acceptable.

How can we begin to heal mamas so that they can have healthy babies? Through education! Education = Power, and those who are educated about pregnancy become empowered.

Chapter 3
Get Your Mind Right

The Toxic Mind

More and more, women are entering into prenatal care with what I call a "Toxic Mind". As I am interviewing them about their medical histories and current conditions their responses are full of drama and confusion. The numbers of patients with mental disorders is astounding. I am often asking myself, why does every other woman think she is bi-polar, or clinically depressed? What is going on in the world?

If your conversations are full of words like "that bitch", "these niggas", "I ain't no punk", and "they tryin to play me"…you definitely have a Toxic Mind, and no room in it for the development of a healthy baby. In fact, your thoughts will actually harm the baby.

Did you know that every time you think a thought, you produce certain chemicals (hormones) in your brain to accompany that thought? For example, picture yourself in an argument, yelling and screaming about absolutely nothing important. Think about how you feel (physically) in the midst of that argument. Your immediate reaction is anger. Along with that anger is a gush of angry chemicals (hormones) produced by the brain, and traveling through the blood. These chemicals are what make you actually 'feel' angry. Guess who else is exposed to these angry feelings. You guessed it. You are right in the midst of producing an angry and confrontational baby.

The next time you find yourself saying any of the words above, pause, and think about how you feel. I guarantee that you don't feel good. Those are all stress causing words and phrases, and you are much too intelligent to carry on that kind of conversation, whether it is in your mind, or out loud.

Know Your Value

We cannot accomplish anything amazing in life until we know our value. Why? Because when we don't know our value, we don't know what to ask for, or how to set our expectations. As a result, we accept less from ourselves, and from others.

Have you ever been around a very confident person, who absolutely knows their value? The energy that confident people exude is powerful.

Most women tell me that they know their value, but when I ask them to tell me their value they are stuck. It is such a huge question, and to be honest, most of us, myself included, where never taught our value as children.

If I ask you your value, what I am asking you is what your expectations are for yourself, as well as your expectations of how others interact and communicate with you. People who know their value set high expectations for themselves and those around them. How you see yourself dictates your behavior, how others see you, and the respect that you are given. Respect should be just a minimum.

For example:

Do you allow people to address you in a disrespectful manner? Do your friends (men and/or women) refer to you as a "Bitch"? This is a common practice in our communities. On any given day when walking down the street you may witness groups of young girls casually referring to one another in degrading terms such as Bitch. "Bitch, that's what I'm talking about." When you witness this, do you stop and correct them? Do you accept whatever answer someone gives you because you are too afraid to ask for what you want? Do people carry on with inappropriate conversations around you?

If you answer yes to any or all of these questions, you do not know your true value.

***

Real Life Story

A 14 year old patient came in for her first visit. She was 27 weeks pregnant, and through interviewing her, I learned that she was pregnant by a 24 year-old man. This was a patient who had admitted to being molested by two different men as a child (when even younger than 14).

She got very angry with me when I told her that she is still being molested. "No I am not" she said with attitude. I told her that the 24 year-old that is having sex with her is definitely molesting her, and that it is a crime.

I asked for his contact information, and told her that I planned on reporting him so that he wouldn't have the opportunity to molest anyone else's 14 year-old. Her response, "He loves me, and I have already put *him* through too much.

I couldn't believe it. Here he is committing a crime by impregnating her. Do you think she knows her value? Of course not…

And sadly, when I tried to explain to her that she was much too valuable to be giving away her body to a 24 year-old man who should be in college or working at a job, dating women his own age, she got angry. She did not return.

***

Be careful who you lay with

In today's society, women sleep with men too quick. What is expected in return? Nothing! There was a time when a man was required to produce evidence before he could win the company of a woman. What was the evidence you may wonder? Evidence of his faith and character, evidence of his income and work ethic, and evidence that he loved his mama. Are these things important? Of course!

Culturally, blacks have always known that a good man loves God and his mama. In the not so distant past, a man was expected and required to financially take care of his family. He had to work, and work hard. In contrast, today women are taking care of men.

Women are giving men their bodies for the least of reasons. "He is cute! I like his car, girl, he got money…" Yet, the meaningful questions never get asked. Is he respectful? Does he have children? Does he take care of his children? Does he work? Is he religious? These questions don't even get asked. It seems that women today don't value themselves enough to care about the evidence, or maybe it's that the less women and men know about one another the easier it is to have casual sex.

When I asked my 19 year-old daughter about casual sex, and why it is so easy, she told me that sex is an expectation today. Sex is an expectation for the simplest of a date. For example, a girl meets a cute guy in the morning, he tells her that he will pick her up this evening for a date, they go to the movies, and after they have sex. No love, no commitment, hell—she doesn't even know his last name. There is something really disturbing about this picture. As my daughter says, "it is just the way it has become; sometimes it is peer pressure, because everyone is having sex."

What happens when the woman who just had sex after that first date ends up pregnant? Pregnant by a man that she doesn't even (really) know...What will be the consequences to her and the baby? The man has no attachment to her, or the baby...How will she convince him to stay? Will he love the baby?

The product of many of these casual relationships is a baby. A baby produced by two people who barely knew one another, may be undereducated, may be unemployed, may have mental disorders, may use drugs, may have sexually transmitted diseases, and may be ignorant to all the elements necessary to produce productive, secure and loved children.

How can I come to this conclusion? Easily! Look at the black communities of today. It is not hard to see that our community has been destroyed by crack cocaine and other drugs, gang violence, fatherless households, incarcerated males, a hip-hop mentality, low self-esteem, and other socio-economic ills.

We have to realize that two crazy people produce crazy! Two dysfunctional people produce dysfunction! It is simple mathematics...

How can we as women expect a man that we barely know to father a child for the next 18 years? I mean he bears as much responsibility as us, but whether or not he assumes responsibility is a 'crap shoot.'

Many men today are shaped by the pictures in rap videos. Mentally, they believe that the more money they have, the more women they can have sex with. The nicer their cars, the better women will think about them. The more 'thuggish' they look and act, the more women they will attract…Women, are you proving them right? Are you dating a man whose underwear show through his pants? Is that acceptable to you?

I often remind my daughters of the power they have as females. Men do things to impress women. That gives women an enormous amount of power. Men wear their pants low because they think women like it. Men buy shiny cars to attract women. Men try to act "cool" to impress women. Imagine how women could change communities if they all decided against casual sex. Communities would improve instantly.

I can't tell you how many pregnant women that I see in the clinic who are clueless about who the father of their baby is. You may think it only happens on the Maury Povich show, but the truth is, it is very common. This means that women are not only sleeping with one unworthy man, who they probably barely know, but even more. As a result, we are often in the clinic performing ultrasounds so that we can date pregnancies, and find out down to the week, who's the daddy.

***

Real Life Story

A patient came into the clinic for Orientation. She wasn't scheduled to see the clinician on this day, but while seeing the health educator for the first time, she mentioned that she had been using drugs throughout her pregnancy. The health educator asked me to speak with the patient about several of her concerns.

Upon further interview I learned that the patient had been in jail during most of her pregnancy. She believed that she was 27 weeks pregnant based on her last menstrual period, but she hadn't received an ultrasound to confirm this.

Because of her drug use during the pregnancy, and the fact that she was entering care late, I ordered an ultrasound. The ultrasound technician determined that the patient was 20 weeks pregnant, not 27 weeks.

The patient's response was alarming.

"Damn, so this is Ray's baby. Is there anyway this ultrasound could be wrong, because it is possible that three men could be the father of my baby, and if I am 20 weeks it is Ray."

I couldn't help but think "Is she serious?" Unfortunately, these situations happen all too often

***

Do you know how dangerous it is to give your body to just any man? Women have something that is sacred—a womb (uterus). We bring new life into the world. President Barack Obama came via a woman's womb, as did his wife Michelle. Who did you produce? The womb is something special, yet more and more, we give it away for free, or because some man took us to the shop and got our nails done.

Why is it important to protect our womb? Why is it important to discriminate against who we give ourselves to (sexually and mentally)? Well, we have to protect against the unwanted result of sexual irresponsibility…baby daddies, single-mamas, broken homes, and fallen communities.

The Science of Mating
There is a science to mating. One that is still practiced today in many cultures, often referred to as arranged marriages. There was a time that I looked down on this concept thinking that it was an oppressive practice, but now I have a new appreciation for this practice. You live, and learn.

What do I mean when I say that there is a science to mating? Well, when two people unite and make a baby, many factors become relevant. Was daddy lazy, or crafty? Was mom educated, or ignorant? Was mom or dad (or both) using drugs? Were mom and dad in love? What about his family? Is he responsible? Has he been incarcerated? The answers to these questions and many more will matter and will affect your life in the future.

I am almost jealous that there are still cultures that care enough about their children to interfere. In the black community today, young women have (almost) no one to talk to about relationships. Not if they expect to get sound advice. My experience at the clinic is that the mamas of my patients are as crazy as their daughters. I literally see 40 year-old women with worse behavior than their 17 year-old daughters.

My Own Baby Daddy Experience

When I was 16 years old, I was hanging out with an older sister of mine in Valencia Gardens, a public housing project in San Francisco. This super cute guy passed by in a Cherry Apple Red Mustang, trimmed in Gold. He was blasting Slick Rick's song, A Bedtime Story. I asked my sister who he was, and I remember the excitement in my sister's voice as she told me, "ooh girl, he got money, you need to hook-up with him…I will introduce you to him" As a result of that introduction, 20 years later I have an adult daughter by a man that I never loved, and quite frankly never knew well enough to justify having his baby. Oh yeah, but his car was cute.

The "so-called" relationship between the father of my baby and I was filled with madness, stress, and sorrow. It was like a horrible cycle…me chasing him, him cheating, me questioning him, him lying, him in jail, me accepting collect calls and visiting him…dysfunctional as hell. In fact, that is what it was, HELL.

After the birth of my daughter, life was hard for me. Despite the fact that her father was dealing drugs, and had plenty of money, he wasn't truly taking care of his child. In his immature mind, he thought that buying an occasional pair of tennis shoes, or the new hot wheels car was being a daddy. I would often remind him that our daughter eats everyday, not just once a month.

In reflection, I can't think of one thing that made the father of my daughter worthy of a prize like me. He was unemployed; he was undereducated, and irresponsible. Most of all, he didn't recognize or appreciate my value. Sadly, I didn't recognize my value. This made the relationship doomed.

What I needed was someone to tell me the truth. The truth was that I was pregnant by a man who didn't love or respect me. Hell, he didn't even love or respect himself. Just like me, he was a victim of the streets. Someone should have told me to sit down, shut-up, and peep game. That it was going to be really hard once the baby came, and the truth was that the father of my daughter wouldn't be there, at least not for long.

The Message

As young women, we waste so much time trying to convince ourselves that a lie is the truth. We've been lied to throughout our entire lives. We know that our relationships are dysfunctional. We know that the men aren't committed to us. We know that they are cheating; the STDs that they are bringing home should be proof enough. Maybe it is embarrassment that causes us to continue living lies and covering for unworthy men.

What do we do? We suffer in silence. We make excuses for men that are not worthy. We know they are not supporting their children, but what do we do? We get two jobs, or work harder in the job that we have, just so that we can be with somebody.

My husband once told me that women make weak men when we make excuses for them. Stop making excuses and put some expectations on your man. If he won't even *try* to meet your expectations, he is not the *one* for you—point blank. If you discover that he is not the *one*, get out of the relationship immediately, before the babies start to come, or at least before another baby comes.

The End of the Baby Daddy Syndrome

There is power in words. That is something that I learned from my aunt. I never liked the way "My Baby Daddy" sounded, so I rarely used it. I would rather just call the father of my daughter by his name.

Calling the father of your baby, "My Baby Daddy", cheapens the relationship between you and him, and him and the baby. It is sabotaging, causing you to desensitize yourself toward his obligations and duties. It disassociates you from him. "Oh, he is (just) my Baby's Daddy." This thinking affects the way that you think about the pregnancy, and ultimately the child.

Saying the words, "My husband" affects you mentally, and in a very different way than saying the words "My Baby Daddy". "My husband" makes you feel secure, loved, and worthy. It produces a very different combination of hormones in your brain that travel directly to your baby, delivering the same feelings of security and love. That is the beginning of having a healthy baby, and family.

Sista, if you are in a relationship with the father of your baby and you are not married, **Get Married**! In fact, demand it! You may say that marriage won't change anything. If he wants to leave he can still leave. You are right, he can leave, but it is definitely not as easy.

If you are in a relationship, but have not made the decision to get married, discuss it immediately. Talk to married elders in the community, and go to (pre) marriage counseling so that you will enter into marriage successfully.

You may say, "I don't need to get married, we've been together forever—like 12 years." That is not the case. There are certain privileges and recognitions that come with marriage, especially when a child is in the picture.

***

Real Life Story

When a friend of mine found out that I was writing this book, she made a special request that I add her story. Why? She wanted to share with sistas that no matter how long you've been in a relationship, when you are not married, the relationship is incomplete.

After having her third baby, and while still in the hospital, the nurses put the identification wristband around the baby's wrist. She noticed that the wristband said Baby X, which was her last name. She called it to the attention of the nurses, because the last name of her baby, like her other two babies, is the last name of her boyfriend, (not her). She explained to them that her and her boyfriend have been together for 13 years, and requested that they change the last name on the wristband. The nurses explained to her that because they were not married, the wristband had to remain in her last name.

To this day, it bothers her that the wristband was not changed to reflect her boyfriends last name, and she admits that as she thinks about it more, there are other situations similar to this that have affected her no matter how long her relationship.

Her advice to you, GET MARRIED. She is planning to be married this fall.

***

Do not let a man continue to lay with you without commitment. It is not healthy. It is not building family or community. Most of all, you deserve more and your baby deserves more. Make that man your husband, and you be his wife. That is definitely 'what's up'

In contrast, if you are in a relationship and it is going nowhere, you have a hard decision to make. If you are in a relationship with a man who is not in a relationship with you—end that relationship. Get that man out of the way, so that you can make way at a later time for a man that will love, respect and MARRY you. You are worth it.

Can I guarantee that your marriage will last? No. Is it worth it to try? Yes. And when I say try that is what I mean. Don't give up so easily. If you get married, fight to make it work. Fight for yourself, and fight for you children.

"Keep a Nigga" Babies

I know that some of these terms sound too crazy to be true, but I didn't make them up. Another phenomenon in our communities is the belief that if we become pregnant, we will be able to keep our men. This is so false, and in truth, you know it is false when you try. If you can't keep your man without the addition of a baby, you definitely will not be able to keep him with the addition of a baby. A baby only complicates things when you are not in a committed relationship. What is the outcome? A Baby Daddy, who like before the baby, is uninterested and irresponsible. Now you have to beg him for more than attention. You have to beg him for diapers, formula and the love of his child.

***

Exercise I

Write two paragraphs identifying your dream husband.

In the first paragraph, describe him…What does he look like? How is his behavior? Where does he work? What about his family? How does he treat you? Does he believe in God? If so, what is his religion? Etc…

In paragraph two, explain **why** all of these characteristics and qualities are important to you?

Exercise II

Compare your current partner to your dream husband.

On a piece of paper, make two columns. In the first column write Pros and in the other column write Cons.

For each of your expectations and desires (identified in Exercise I) that your partner meets, list it in the Pros column. For each expectation and desire that your current partner doesn't meet, list it in the Cons column.

How does your mate weigh? Are there more Pros or Cons? Review the results based on your expectations and WHY they were important to you. If the results show that you are in a relationship that can grow, use this exercise as a discussion tool with your partner, explaining to him your expectations, and why they are important to you.

Note: You should never have to explain to a man why it is important for him to work and strive to support his family. He already knows that. It is part of his Nature. If you find yourself having to explain this, this man is not interested in you. Men who love their families will strive to support them.

If your paper is full of Cons, you have some decisions to make, and fast.

***

A Sad Observation
Although all races of women are battling the Baby Mama Epidemic, no group of women has been as affected as black women. While providing prenatal care I have made an interesting observation. At first, I thought it was a co-incidence, but as the days, weeks, months and years have passed, I cannot deny it.

- Most black women come to their prenatal visits alone, or with other women (friends/family).
- Most Latino and white women come with their partner.
- Ironically, when white women are pregnant by black men, the men come to the prenatal visits.

My question is why? Why don't black men support their women in pregnancy and childbirth? From my experiences as a midwife, and the stories that I have heard from women, I have formed my own conclusion. It is because black men and women are not in healthy relationships. Rather we have Baby Daddies. We met somebody, he was cute, and whoops, I'm pregnant. No commitment at all. No requirements on the man and no expectations. What do we end up with? A Baby Daddy! Even worse, a baby daddy who you hardly know, and who probably is somebody else's baby's daddy too.

***

Exercise I

Write down three ways that you will ask your partner (or the father of your baby) to accompany you to your next three visits.

Next, write down why it is important (to you) that he accompanies you.

Exercise II

On one piece of paper write down your response to your partner (or the father of your baby) if he agrees to accompany you. This response should be pleasant, and should include why you appreciate his presence.

On another piece of paper write down what your response will be if he disagrees to accompany you. On this paper include facts such as black babies die three times more than white babies, and that black men rarely accompany their partners to visits. Also, tell him how it makes you feel when he doesn't accompany you to visits (alone, embarrassed, etc...) See if reasoning makes a difference.

If he is not interested in accompanying you to any of your visits for any reason other than work, this should be a "Red Flag".

***

Chapter 4
Change Your Lifestyle

Stressed Out!

It breaks my heart to see the numbers of women who come into the clinic in tears. The reason is stress; the realization that things are just not "right" in their life. Usually, it is the uncertainty about their relationship with the father of the baby, or financial struggles.

Stress is a physical, mental and/or emotional response to events. It causes bodily or mental tension. The result of long term stress is sometimes manifested in weight gain, high blood pressure, migraine headaches, heart attack, stroke and other diseases.

Why do black women have so much stress? Although some of our stress comes from the pressures of everyday society, I would argue that we are responsible for bringing most of the stress into our lives because of the poor choices that we make as women

An unplanned pregnancy can be tremendously stressful on its own, but when adding the additional stressor of a Baby Daddy instead of a husband, it can be detrimental. For example, if your partner does not want the baby, but you do, that can cause stress. Or if your finances aren't where they should be that is definitely a stressor. When you add the addition of a new baby, it gets even more stressful. If you have other children that you are caring for, without the adequate resources or support, it can also be stressful, especially if you aren't with the father of the other children. Then there is the question of whether or not the father of this baby will stay with you and help raise the baby.

These are all questions that should have been answered before conception. Ideally, they are answered in a conversation that you have with your husband before planning or conceiving a baby. But…just because that wasn't the case doesn't mean that you can't turn a negative into a positive and work to eliminate as much stress as possible.

To eliminate the stressors identified above arrange time to talk with your partner. As soon as you learn about the pregnancy, sit down and discuss your plan of action. All too often women come into the clinic disappointed about their partner's response to the pregnancy, or actions throughout the pregnancy. Several women have even come in suicidal because their partners have left them. These are usually women that have not communicated their expectations to their partners, so they are both walking in the blind.

If you expect your partner to provide half of the rent money, you have to tell him. If you expect him to buy the weekly groceries, you have to communicate with him. You can't expect him to read your mind. Just because you believe that something is reasonable, you can't assume that your partner will. Sometimes we want people to do the right thing just because we think it is right. Then we become disappointed because they didn't do it.

No where in the equation did we communicate our expectations to them, so we can't hold them accountable for the failure without giving them an opportunity to do right by us.

You may think that you shouldn't have to tell your partner to pay half the rent, or to buy the weekly groceries, and I agree. However, you are not taking into account how this man was raised, what he values, and even whether or not he has seen a functional relationship. But, because these issues were not discussed before sex, they have become difficult issue to discuss after sex, when emotions are entangled into the mix.

So much of our stress could be eliminated with honest communication. Even when you are not with the father of your baby, you still must communicate your expectations to him so that he won't leave the burden with you. He is not excused from parenting his child. There is much to discuss, and by gaining clarity about each topic, you will relieve a tremendous amount of stress.

Some of the key points that you will need clarity about are:

- How much money he will provide monthly to support your baby? (When you discuss this issue, have some reasonable expectations. For example, diapers cost X amount, and the baby will need X amount of diapers monthly. This means that you need X amount of money from him)…

- How much time he will commit to spending with his baby?
- If he is able to assist with childcare so that you can attend school or work?
- What will be your level and mode of communication after the baby?

You cannot make appropriate plans to mother a child with minimal stress, until you agree on acceptable answers to the questions above.

As we have been identifying, there is a tremendous amount of stress in the daily lives of many women. As midwives, we tell women to decrease stress, but if your entire life is stressful, stress becomes a normal factor of daily life, and hard to identify.

In relation to the identification of daily stressors I have provided some exercises.

***

Exercise I: Define stress

Write a paragraph explaining what stress means to you. Identify where you have obvious stress in your life, and then explain why you have allowed that stress to continue, and how you can eliminate that the stress.

Exercise II: 5-day Journal

For the next week, keep a journal. In the journal you are going to keep a diary of your daily activities (from waking up, to going to sleep). When you have completed the journal, go through each page and highlight all of the events that were stressful. On a separate piece of paper write each event that caused stress, and what you can do to eliminate that stress from your routine.

This activity will help you identify the stressful events that might not be so obvious.

***

Sistas' Gonna Work It Out

Women don't like other women for no sensible reason. It is something we learn in society. It is baffling how we as women don't trust one another, but we are quick to trust an unworthy man. Even after he has proven that he is not trustworthy. Why?

As a result of our general distrust of one another, we haven't learned to confide in each other, depend on each other, or to ask for help when we need it. Instead, we would rather suffer, and wait on a man that we know is not going to come through. Amazing!

Sistas, get to know, and befriend women in your community. Form a tight-knit group of like-minded, trustworthy sistas that you can socialize and commune with on a regular basis.

***

Real Story

I have a friend that I admire greatly. She is an African American, OB-Gyn doctor in California. A while back she shared one of her *lessons learned* while in medical school. It was the value of asking for help when you need it.

This woman grew up in a poor community in West Oakland, always wanting to be a doctor. When she finally went to medical school she was a single mother of three. Things were tough in medical school, no surprises, but sooner than later, things got really difficult. She contemplated coming home, which turned out NOT to be an option.

Finally she realized that she needed help, but struggled with asking for help, because it is taboo in our communities. It wasn't until she identified other single mothers at her medical school who were in the same situation, that she realized the value of those women, and the value of asking for help. They formed a network, and they alternated providing childcare.

This relationship was one of those that helped her get through medical school, return home and serve her community.

How has your distrust of other women been holding you back from progress?

***

Get an Education

You cannot support a baby on welfare. Nor can you support a baby with a minimum-wage job. If you think you can, you will definitely bring some stress into your life.

The purpose of welfare is to help women (and families) out when times are hard. Times should only be hard for a season. If times are always hard for you then something is wrong. Welfare is a trap, and if you let it, it will keep you broke.

Now is an excellent time to get an education. If you did not graduate from high school, enroll in an adult education program. If you did complete high school enroll in college or a vocational program. Learn a skill.

Being that you are going to be the first teacher of your new baby, you are going to have to increase your knowledge base. Education is a must for you if you plan on getting a decent job that will pay you a living wage. Take advantage of this time and just do it.

You will find that the more education you acquire, the less tolerant you will be of foolishness, and foolish people.

You *Can* Turn a 'Ho' into a Housewife

Every female who grew up in the 'hood' has heard the saying, "you can't turn a 'ho' into a housewife". What did they mean?

To put it in straight words, men don't want women that have been (sexually) with everyone in the community. Nor do they want women who say that they are not promiscuous, but they wear the uniform (dressed in slinky, tasteless clothes). It reminds me of a line from a Lauren Hill Song, That Thing. "Showing off your ass cause you thinking it's a trend." Guess what, it's not! No self respecting woman would leave her home wearing low-rider jeans and a G-String (showing). This is a clear indication of low-self esteem. Clearly you need attention, but is this the way you want to ask? What type of attention do you think this will attract?

I see so many women in the clinic who are crying for attention—8 months pregnant wearing a tank top and booty shorts. Why? Do you think that a real man wants the mother of his child dressed like this? Even worse, dressed like this while pregnant.

Men don't take you seriously when all they see is your ass. Why? Because ALL they see is your ass. Especially in the Hip-Hop Generation, you remind them of some video vixen that they saw on the new Lil' Wayne video—only good for one thing. What man wants to be out and about, when he realizes that all his *'boys'* have been with his *'girl'*?

You will not catch your husband like this. What you will catch at most is a 'Baby Daddy', or at least a sexually transmitted disease. If that doesn't cause enough embarrassment and pain, you will be left with memories of a one-night stand, or being used (and abused).

Men talk. What do they talk about? Women! Don't think that you and he will be the only two who know about your night of casual sex. By the next morning all his friends, and some of yours will know.

Men respect women who demand and command respect. That is the woman that they will strive to please. Be that woman! Men disrespect women who disrespect themselves by giving *it'* up too fast, and to too many men. Be respectable, be respectful and be self-respecting. It will reduce a lot of your stress.

No One Wants to Hear a Woman Cussing and Carrying-On in Public

You get back from the Universe what you put in. If you run around the community acting like a savage, you end up with stress.

Have you ever been at home in the daytime and you turn on the Maury Povich Show? It is appalling. There are actually women who go on television to learn who the father of their baby is. Even more appalling, they are not embarrassed. Then when they find out whether or not the man that they brought on the show is the father, instead of being humble so that they can work out a relationship for the benefit of the child, what do they do? They start screaming at him, "Now! I told yo ass!"…jumping around calling him names, and acting a complete fool. Sistas, where is the dignity?

If I hear another loud mouth woman on a talk show embarrassing herself. Or some woman talking on her cell phone or to her buddies loud and disrespectful in public, I am going to scream. The rest of the world is not interested in your conversation. We don't care who you are mad at, or who you are dating. It looks awful. If you think this behavior impresses someone, it does not! People are laughing at you—not with you.

Learn to think before you speak. Listen to how people that you admire communicate. Would you hear Oprah Winfrey, or Michelle Obama using curse words in public? Then why are you? You know it is not right, yet you don't have the strength to reject that behavior.

***

Real Life Story

I was seeing a patient for the first time. It wasn't her first time in the clinic, only her first time seeing me. As I was asking her some questions about her pregnancy, and writing in her chart, she asked me, "Are you part Nigga?" I could not believe that she had asked me that question, so I turned toward her and asked, "Excuse me?"…She asked me again, without stuttering, "Are you part Nigga?"

I almost thought that I was on Candid Camera, because no one had ever asked me anything so inappropriate. I couldn't help but think, "Is this what we've become?"

If you only get one chance to make a First Impression, she didn't do too well. How would you do?

You may be thinking that this is an extreme example, but I would argue that it is not. I may not hear the same words, but I see patient after patient with offensive behavior and conversation.

***

As women, mothers, or soon-to-be mothers, it is urgent that we relearn the proper way to behave, and communicate. After all, women are the first teachers. What will you teach (offer) your baby? Surely it is not loud-talking and gum-popping. When you act inappropriately in public, it is offensive to others and it makes you look ignorant.

There is a way to conduct ourselves at home and abroad, both personally, and when conducting business. The sooner women learn the proper way, the more successful we will become. You don't conduct business while texting or talking on your cell phone, listening to your IPOD, and definitely not with an attitude. People are looking at us and thinking, "What happened to them?" There was a time when blacks had stellar manners. To be in public and acting other than dignified was not acceptable.

If we were honest with ourselves, the root of it is low self-esteem. We are looking for love and admiration, but no one ever taught us how to get positive attention.

There is no way to change your life without changing bad behavior. What better time than during pregnancy? You are about to bring a new life into the world. Don't bring a new life into the world with the same bad behavior.

By changing your behavior for the best, you reduce stress immediately. You begin to have healthy relationships, and people start to show you respect.

Go Tell It on the Mountain

This is definitely a Facebook Generation, and fittingly we publish all of our business online. Why? Half of the information we post is embarrassing.

Facebook is for networking and keeping in touch with peers. Not for showing your ass, and how ignorant you act when you leave home. Stop telling all your business online, and leave something for the imagination. Before a person gets to know you, they already have an idea of who you are- you posted it on Facebook. When you post something online it is public. Remember that.

Yes, Marijuana is a Drug

I can't quantify how many women I see throughout my clinic days who are surprised when I inform them that their urine screen has come back positive for Marijuana, a.k.a. weed. To my amazement, women seem to think that if they smoke weed, it doesn't count toward substance abuse. Their excuse, "Oh, that's just weed. I have to smoke weed because it helps me with my nausea and to keep food down". Guess what, you don't get to smoke weed because you have nausea. Many women experience nausea, and they don't smoke Marijuana.

Links are being identified between Marijuana use during pregnancy and behavioral problems in the children that were exposed to Marijuana use in the womb. Do you want to be the mama who has to go to your child's school once a week because he or she can't act right? All because you couldn't stop smoking weed when you were pregnant? It feels right now, but is it worth years and years of struggle and sadness?

Marijuana is a drug, straight up! Using Marijuana during pregnancy exposes your baby to dangerous chemicals, and can affect your baby's development. If that information isn't compelling enough, you should also know that Child Protective Services may get involved in your care when you consistently test positive for Marijuana use, and they absolutely **will** get involved in your care if you test positive for certain other drugs.

Sit back and think about the way you feel when you are high. Think about the terms associated with being high. Stoned! Stuck on Stupid! Bombed…Remember, there is power in words. What you feel, your baby feels.

My advice: Love yourself and your baby too much to succumb to drug use. There is NO good in it, and our communities have been destroyed since the strategic introduction of drugs.

Think the Right Thoughts

If all you listen to are songs like Birthday Sex and Lollypop, you will never accomplish anything. These are just the type of songs that bring our thinking down, keeping lowly, savage thoughts on the brain.

We learned earlier that the thoughts that we think create chemical reactions in our brain and when women are pregnant, these thoughts travel through the blood to the baby.

What chemicals do you think we create when we are cursing, or watching inappropriate rap videos?

Try to be mindful of your thoughts. Are you always sad and crying? Are you always angry and arguing? The result could be a 'cry-baby', or a baby that is confrontational. Is it worth it?

By controlling your thoughts, not only will you help your baby, but you will also help yourself. Your life cannot begin to change until you change the way you think.

Surround Yourself with the Right People

We judge people by the company they keep. If you are hanging around with a bunch of bar hopping, promiscuous, scandalous women, then why wouldn't we think you are the same? If you were a scholar, you would hang around with scholars. Drug dealers hang with drug dealers. Pimps hang with prostitutes...It is common sense.

You cannot make a change for the better if you continue to hang around with people who are not (also) trying to change. They will hold you down.

Have you ever heard the saying 'Fake It Till You Make It'? That stands true today. Until you get where you want to be, you should be rehearsing on a regular basis. Life is a Dress Rehearsal. Be found rehearsing where you want to be, instead of regressing into bad behaviors.

***

Exercise I

Write three paragraphs explaining a person, or persons, that you admire, what they do, and the company that they keep. For example, if you admire your aunt because she is very successful, then write down her name, why you believe she is successful, what type of friends she has, and where you could meet similar friends.

***

Personal Testimony

When I was younger I had lots of friends, but in reflection I found that my friends were always fighting, causing confusion, and scheming in some way. They didn't work—they hustled, and it was exhausting.

Our behavior never attracted anything positive, and the result of our behavior was generally stressful.

Several years after the birth of my oldest daughter I made the decision to change my lifestyle. I identified some people that I admired. They were mostly community activist, so I started to attend community meetings. I befriended some of them, and today we still communicate.

If you were to look at my circle of friends today, they are working professionals, educated, and responsible. They all have some strength that is attracting. They are a reflection of what I respect.

***

Chapter 5
Get Your 'Health' On

Toxic Body

Starting your pregnancy in good health will help you to end the pregnancy with a healthy baby. Too many black women today walk into their initial prenatal visit with layers of health concerns, physically and mentally.

More and more patients are presenting with obesity, diabetes, hypertension, hepatitis, liver disease and kidney problems. We eat the wrong foods, and resist regular doctor visits.

Being overweight presents a significant risk during pregnancy. It can cause babies to get stuck during delivery, or to grow too large. Obesity is an epidemic in our community.

You Are What You Eat

How many times have you heard 'You Are What You Eat' growing up? Guess what, it is truer now than ever. With food quality on the decline, less time available to make healthy meals, and the increase in stress levels, women are quickly becoming overweight.

Not only does food affect our weight, but it affects our thoughts. Today, meat is full of hormones. Cows, chickens and pigs are being injected with hormones so that they can grow faster and larger. What do you think happens to people when they eat meat that has been injected with hormones? The hormones transfer to people. Then we notice our little girls developing breast at 8 years-old, and starting their menstrual cycles at 9.

The way that an animal is killed has influence on the hormones in the meat that we eat. In ancient cultures there is a proper way to slaughter an animal. In America, they are simply killed. If the animal isn't killed properly, and it is scared when it dies, it has harmful hormones present in its body. Then, we eat the animal, hormones and all. We wonder why we are always scared.

Pork is a filthy animal. Pigs do not sweat, and the result is a salty taste when you eat Pork. The salty taste is because of the toxins that couldn't escape through the sweat glands. Not to mention that pigs will eat anything. Why don't we love ourselves enough to refrain from eating something so filthy? Sometimes our older relatives will mention that they ate pig for 80 years, and they are still alive. My argument is not the length of your life, but the quality of your life. Will you be happy just living at 80, but not being mobile? Or having heart disease? Protect the quality of your life.

We only have one body, and as hard as it will be, when you start to change your life, you have to address your health. Food and health have a direct relationship.

Your First Prenatal Visit

You can expect to have a complete physical at your initial prenatal visit. Depending on the gestational age of your baby (how many weeks pregnant you are), you may have your abdomen measured and listen to your baby's heartbeat. A vaginal exam, bi-manual exam, and pap smear will also be done at this visit.

The initial prenatal visit is very important as it gives clinicians the opportunity to identify general health issues that may become problematic during your pregnancy. For example, it is at this visit that we listen to your heart and lungs. We also do a Pap Smear to check your cervical health and whether or not you have been exposed to certain sexually transmitted diseases that are problematic during pregnancy. The results of this visit provide us with an opportunity to treat any identified problems, assuming that they are treatable.

Throughout the remainder of your prenatal visits, we will continue to monitor the health of your baby and offer recommended screenings. You can also expect to have an ultrasound so that we can look at the anatomy and growth of the baby.

Knowledge is Power

Prenatal care is crucial to having a healthy baby. Women are waiting to receive prenatal care until their 7th, 8th and even 9th months. Why? You have missed the most informative screening tests and the comprehensive ultrasound at 20 weeks. This ultrasound evaluates your baby's anatomy, and evaluates the baby's growth in comparison to the baby's gestational age. Most importantly you have missed some valuable educational time.

Just so you are aware, when you show up late in your pregnancy for prenatal care, 'Red Flags', go up. We are wondering where you've been. Something in your life has been holding your attention, other than the baby. Was it drugs? Was it an abusive relationship? Denial? There is something there, and we know it.

Entering into prenatal care early gives you the opportunity to learn valuable information about things that can hurt, and help your baby's development. It also gives clinicians the opportunity to offer you many important tools, and access to screening tests.

Urinary Tract Infections (bladder infections) and Bacteria Vaginosis (a vaginal infection) have been linked to preterm labor. These conditions can be easily identified and treated with regular prenatal care. Chlamydia and other sexually transmitted diseases can cause serious problems for your new baby; again, with early identification we can treat these diseases so that you can have a healthy baby.

Typically, the women that enter care late are the women with the most problems and as a result, we end up spending all our time trying to order medications, tests and other procedures that could have been addressed early on.

Despite whatever reason(s) that you are running from prenatal care, most of us are not interested in having your baby taken from you. We simply want to help you to address the risky behavior that may lead to the involvement of Child Protective Services, and eventually your child being taken away.

Use the resources available, and make the changes.

***

Chapter 6
Mission Accomplished! Your Healthy Baby

Now that you are empowered with the information necessary to BEGIN your transformation toward parenthood, let's discuss some ways to keep your new baby healthy.

Another Sad Observation
- Approximately 95% of my Latina patients breastfeed
- Approximately 50% of my white patients breastfeed
- Approximately 1%-3% of my black patients breastfeed

Breastfeeding is the Best
Study, after study has proven that breast milk is best for you, and for your baby. Honestly, if no studies concluded the benefits of breastfeeding, wouldn't it just make sense? Humans produce milk for humans. Cows produce milk for calves. Dogs produce milk for puppies. It just makes sense.

If I told you that breastfeeding your baby could save your baby's life, would that make a difference? Breast milk is full of vitamins, and it boosts the immune system of your baby from birth. Also, breast milk is easier for your baby to digest. Isn't that enough to encourage you to breastfeed?

A challenging time for breastfeeding in the postpartum period is the time between delivery and a patient's 4-6 week postpartum visit. This is the time when women are either successful at breastfeeding, or they give up. Usually, their excuses are that they didn't think they were producing enough milk, or it was too painful.

Once you deliver your baby, if you have any questions about breastfeeding ask your clinician, or ask a WIC Lactation Consultant. Almost always we can work it out, and you can breastfeed.

Breastfeeding Is Not Only About Milk

As mentioned before, many women who stop breastfeeding do so because they don't think they are producing enough milk, or that the baby is not getting full from the milk that they are producing. Why? They believe that because the baby seems to always want to be on the breast, then the baby is not getting enough milk.

This is false. Every time that your baby is at your breast, he or she is not eating. Much of the time your baby is bonding. Just staring at their mama, and using that special one-on-one time to get to know mama better.

Be patient. This is one of the best times and opportunities that you will have to bond with your baby. There is no rush. When the baby wants to suck, the baby will suck. When the baby stops sucking, the baby is bonding. Breast-feeding is comforting to your baby, and is much better than a pacifier.

Breastfeeding also helps mama! It helps your uterus to contract to its normal size, as well as assisting you to return to your pre-pregnancy weight, by burning extra calories.

Do the Right Thing

So now I have told you, in real talk, about the benefits of breastfeeding. If you know that breastfeeding is best, breastfeed. It is time to put the priority on the baby. It is not about you anymore, but about raising a healthy baby.

I spend so much of my time trying to convince moms to do what is best for their babies, when the truth is, as a mom you should want to do what's best—no convincing required.

'A hint to the wise is sufficient'! Are you wise, or igno-rant? Having Integrity, means doing the 'right thing' when no one is looking. I can't love your baby more than you, so do your part and give your baby the love that he or she deserves.

The Party Will Have To Go On Without You

Now that you have a baby, you will have to realize that your social life will not be the same. Don't be that mom who drops her baby off at whose ever house is available. People are crazy today. Protect your baby. You don't know what is going on at that house. They may be getting high, and neglecting to watch your baby, hitting on your baby, or even worse, molesting your baby. Don't risk it. Sacrifice, and stay home from the party. Only allow trusted family and friends to care for your baby.

I always remind my 19 year-old daughter how amazing it is that she is alive today. She was my experimental baby! I was always leaving her with any Tom, Dick or Harry. Thank God nothing (too) bad ever happened to her. I say 'too bad', because who knows what did happen. I was too busy trying to be the life of the party. Don't make the same mistake.

Protect Your Baby from the Ways of the World
During the first several years of your baby's life, they will absorb a tremendous amount of information. Don't teach your baby to curse. Don't have your baby in places that babies shouldn't be. Don't teach your baby how 'to act grown" and talk back. These behaviors are NOT CUTE! In fact, in my opinion this is child abuse.

You have been given a chance in life to do something right! Love and protect your baby. Babies grow up to be adults, and who wants their baby to go through the same struggles that they did. There has been enough of learning by experience. We can no longer afford to expose our children to ignorance.

Many Thanks

Thank you for reading this Guide. I pray that you have accepted the information and experiences that I have provided in the right spirit. Today, we have to speak STRAIGHT WORDS to one another. We can no longer afford to run around confused and ignorant, and definitely not referring to ourselves as Baby Mamas.

This Guide was written with nothing but Love for the Baby Mamas in the community.

Give Thanks.